WELLNESS DIETETIC

TIPS TO EAT WELL AND LIVE HEALTHY

SABAT BEATTO

Copyright 2017, Sabat Beatto
Sidewalk Publisher Inc.
1348 Elder Ave. Bronx, NY 10472
Email: sabeatto@gmail.com

<u>LEGAL NOTICE</u>

The Publisher has strived to be as accurate and complete as possible in the creation of this report, notwithstanding the fact that he does not warrant or represent at any time that the contents within are accurate due to the rapidly changing nature of the Internet.

While all attempts have been made to verify information provided in this publication, the Publisher assumes no responsibility for errors, omissions, or contrary interpretation of the subject matter herein. Any perceived slights of specific persons, peoples, or organizations are unintentional.

In practical advice books, like anything else in life, there are no guarantees of income made. Readers are cautioned to reply on their own judgment about their individual circumstances to act accordingly.

This book is not intended for use as a source of legal, business, accounting or financial advice. All readers are advised to seek services of competent professionals in legal, business, accounting and finance fields.

You are encouraged to print this book for easy reading.

Table Of Contents

Foreword

Where previously most people take health for granted, now most people make a conscious effort to stay healthy. Part of staying healthy is knowing the benefits of exercise, living according to appropriate lifestyle habits, healthy dietary choices and generally keeping stress levels as low as possible. Get all the info you need here.

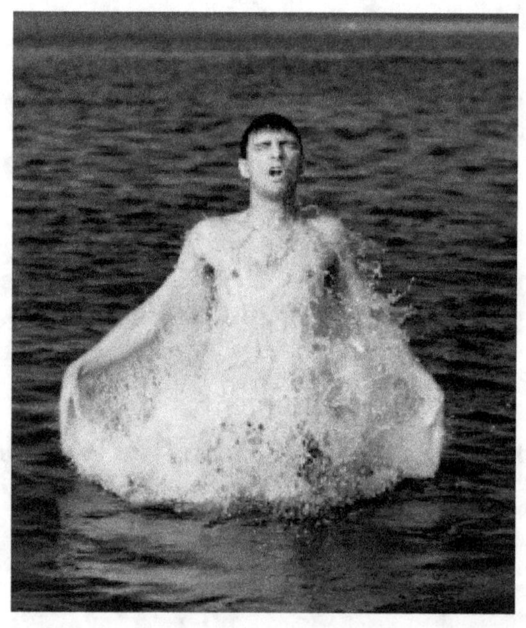

Wellness Dietetic
Amazing Tips To Eat Well And Live Healthy

Chapter 1:

Health Is Wealth

Staying healthy is a very good position to be in, as the opposite of that would be tracking in and out of hospitals with one medical condition or another. This cannot only be depressing but can also severely dent the wallet, as medical bills can be rather expensive to handle. Being able to enjoy life without the burden of popping pills and visiting doctors every so often is definitely a better option to live by.

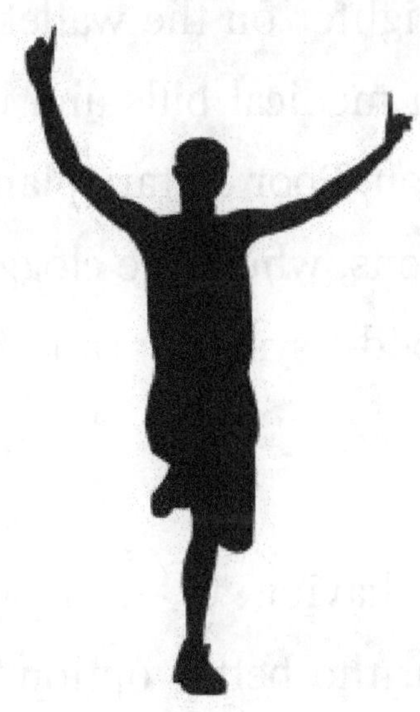

The Basics

Extensive research has shown that many medical conditions are the result of poor eating habits coupled with the lack of consistent exercise and a stress-filled life. Therefore taking the time to seriously address these issues before they turn into problems is one way of keeping healthy.

It would certainly be lighter on the wallet, when the individual is not bogged down with medical bills and the trauma of having to face a terminal condition. Poor dietary plans usually cause less that optimum body conditions, where the clogging, damaging and over working of internal body systems can then contribute to poor health conditions.

Therefore instead of having to deal with the probability of managing poor health, the better option would be to start on a healthy diet plan, a regular exercise regimen and a stress free mindset. Having some knowledge and education on the benefits of healthy living style, will not benefit the individual, if information learnt is not put into practice. As the human body naturally deteriorate as it ages all steps should be taken to ensure the process is not helped along by poor health.

Chapter 2:

Nutrition Is Important

There are a lot of reasons why there are various diets available to the general public, and most of these safer diets are designed around the importance of nutrient content.

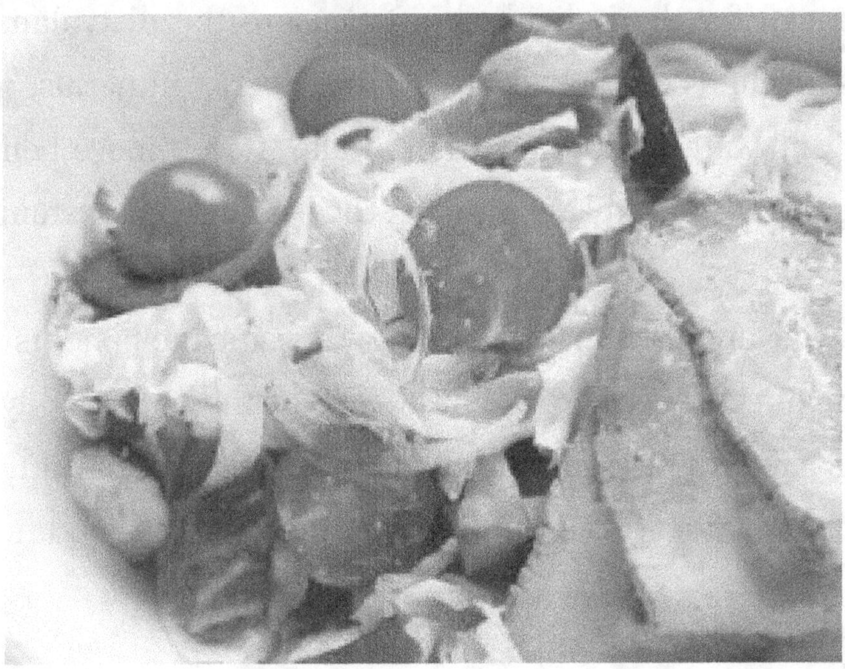

Nutrients

Nutrition is the key factor to a healthy body system which is able to function at its optimum capabilities and also help to maintain an ideal positive overall health condition. One way of ensuring the right nutrition intake is practiced, that the measured amount considered being enough for the individual is to ensure the diet plan includes elements such as carbohydrates, fats, fibers, minerals, proteins, vitamins and water. Good nutrition intake is even more beneficial to specific parts of the body and not just the overall body system.

The following are just some ways of how specific the benefits can be: The heart of course is the essential core of the entire body system; therefore being of such important is needs the special attention so that is cab function at its optimum, thus the need for good nutritional support.

The bones are basically the elements that keep everything together. Here to there is a need for good nutritional support as without optimum bone density and quality the body will experience a lot of connective problems.

Energy for the body is derived from the daily food intake, and there is a need to ensure this food is nutritionally based so that the relevant minerals and vitamins can be dispersed within the system to churn out the necessary energy source for the body's energy needs.

With good nutrition the human body can function at its optimum and basically be able to "last" and with stand any adverse effects the surroundings may throw at it. Often people disregard the importance of good nutrition and this is especially prevalent among the youngsters who seem to think their health in infallible.

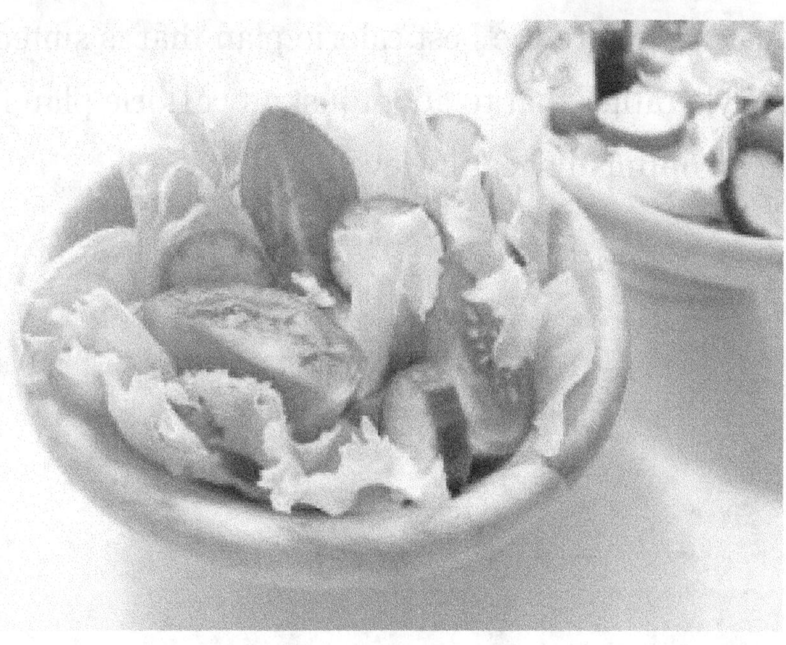

Chapter 3:

Watch Your Calories

Everyone has a different take on the good and bad attributes of having a diet plan low in calorie count. However it would be better for the individual to explore the best calorie plan that is suited for his or her own lifestyle rather that to adopt just any calorie plan in the hope of staying at an optimally healthy level.

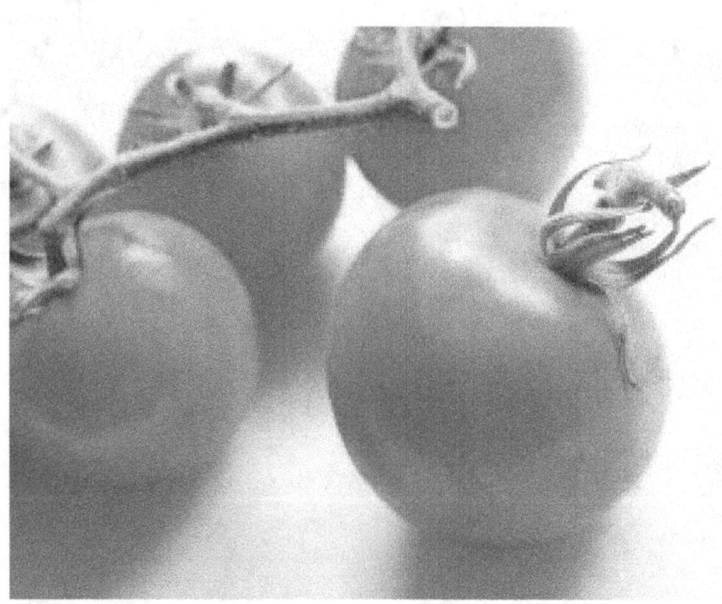

Have A Look

Calories are not bad for the body, in fact they are a necessity as they function as the provider of the energy source for the daily body's needs. The problem lies in the actual intake of calories, where the intake is more than the usage of energy, thus contributing to a high percentage of the unused calorie being stored in the body system and this then contributes to the negative side effects which cause weight gain.

All foods contain calories the only difference is some of these food contain higher amounts of calories than others. The usual measurement of the calorie content would be 1 gram of calorie is broken down into these following contributing measurements – carbohydrate is 4 calories, protein is 4 calories and fat is 9 calories.

Most food product sold will carry the above breakdown for the shopper to have an idea of the calorie content of the item being bought for consumption purposes. Therefore in the quest to watch the calories it would be product to start taking note of the information divulged on the packaging.

A fairly good guideline to go by would be that most green have comparably lower calories content to other foods. Often the sweetened or processed foods have very high calorie content and this is also only slightly less when it comes to the calorie content in meats.

The fattier the meats the higher the calorie content therefore it would be better to opt for as much lean meat intake as possible.

Most children and youngsters don't really need to watch their calorie intake if they practice very active daily routines but for the working adult without any or much physical workouts in the routine watching calories would be something to seriously consider.

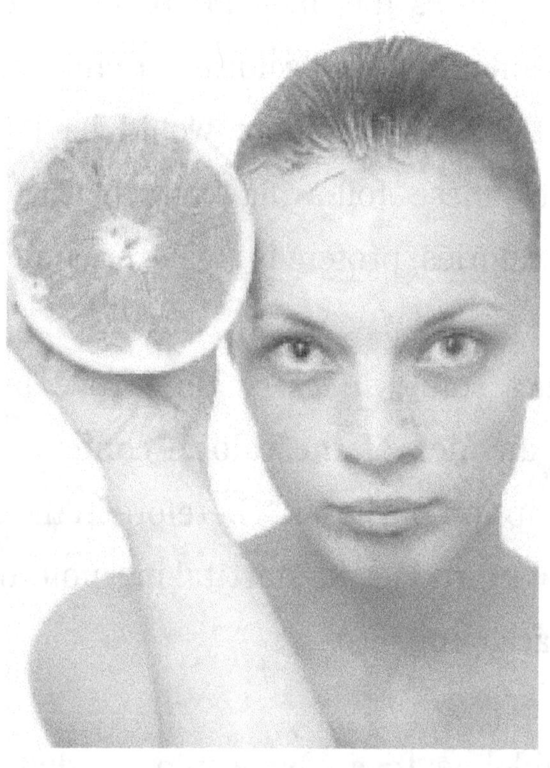

Chapter 4:

Live A Healthy Lifestyle

There are a lot of opinions on how to live a healthy lifestyle, for some it would mean eating only certain foods and following a strict diet plan, for others it would mean a lot of physical exercise and yet for others it would mean living a stress-free lifestyle.

All these have its good attributes and are really quite advantages to follow but nonc can create a healthy lifestyle scenario by itself, ideally it should be a combination of all different positive elements complimenting each other to create the healthy lifestyle.

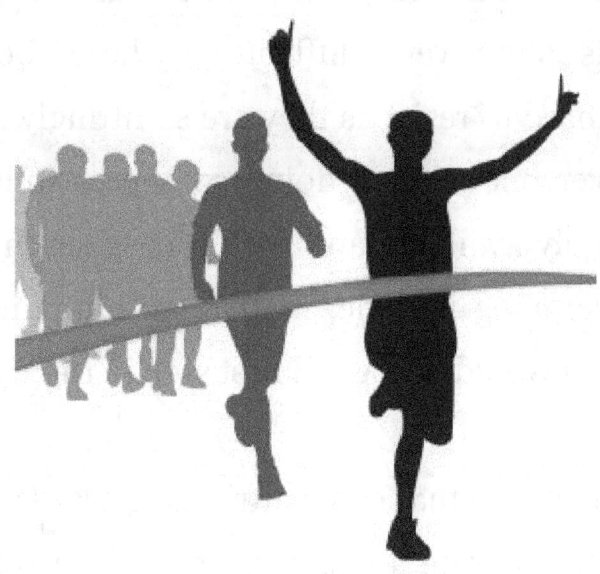

Getting Started

Taking small steps is often a better way to start the healthy lifestyle journey as it does entail some very significant changes. For most people who have go at it all at once, the feeling of being overwhelmed and defeated often causes them to eventually abandon any attempt to pursue a healthy lifestyle regiment.

Making simple adjustments without any drastic eliminating exercises will help to encourage the individual to make further more significant changes as time goes on. These simple steps may include adding more greens and fruits to the current dietary habits.

Cutting down on unhealthy processed snacks is a good step to initiate but is often very difficult as these foods are usually delicious and hard to resist as they are so fittingly named "comfort foods", however one way to doing so successfully is not having such food readily available and within easy reach. The next time the grocery shopping is done, making an effort not to add these items to the cart would be a good first step in the right direction.

Another small change that can contribute towards a better lifestyle would be to incorporate some sort of exercise regiment into the daily or weekly schedule. Although a lot of people give excuses about not having the time for such activities, small changes can be made, such as learning to take the stairs whenever possible as compared to the alternative of using the elevators or escalators.

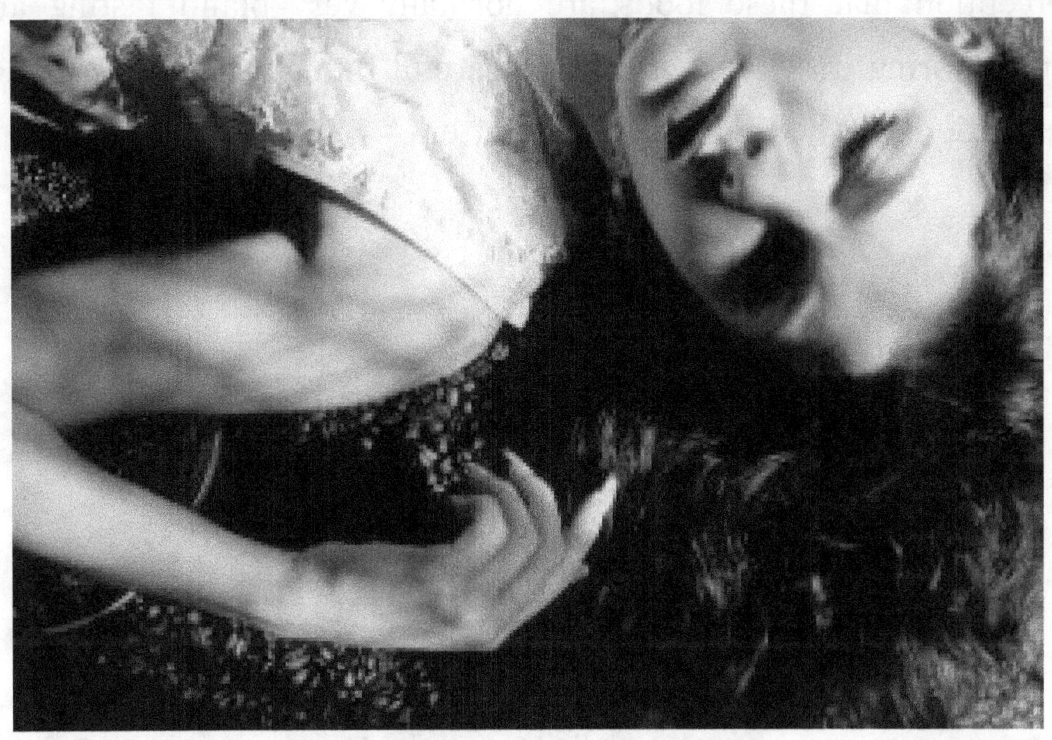

Chapter 5:

Your Food Choices

People often avoid healthy food choices mainly because of the perception that these foods are normally very bland tasting and rather boring. However with some careful thought and efforts such perceptions can be changed for the better.

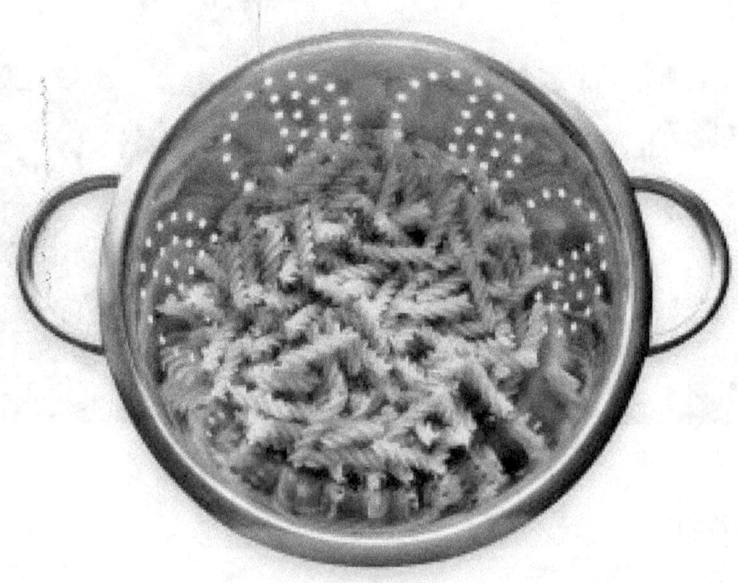

Changing It

Getting children to adapt to healthier food choices can often be a very stressful event, but if such choices were taught to be made from a very early age then the battle will not be an all consuming as imagined. Preparing the healthier food to look and taste better would be the first way to encourage its consumption.

Making conscious decision to reach for healthier options when the opportunity presents itself is a discipline that should be advocated as much as possible. For the more innovative food preparation style there are some who go a step further to actually package the healthier foods to look and feel similar to the unhealthy food choice, an example of which would be presenting celery and carrot sticks in the packaging used to present French fries.

There are also some that package carrot sticks in cigarette boxes and berries in candy packaging. All these are conscious efforts made to play on the mental and visual effects of the individual, in the hope of encouraging the healthier choice being made.

Making other changes gradually such as consuming brown rice and whole-wheat products instead of white products is also another option to look into when making food choices. Having a couple of days dedicated to no meat consumption a week is another good start to make, and this can eventually progress to at least four days a week without meat, but this should not be done in succession as meat consumption is important to the body's needs. Adding more grains and nuts to the diet plan is also another healthy choice to make.

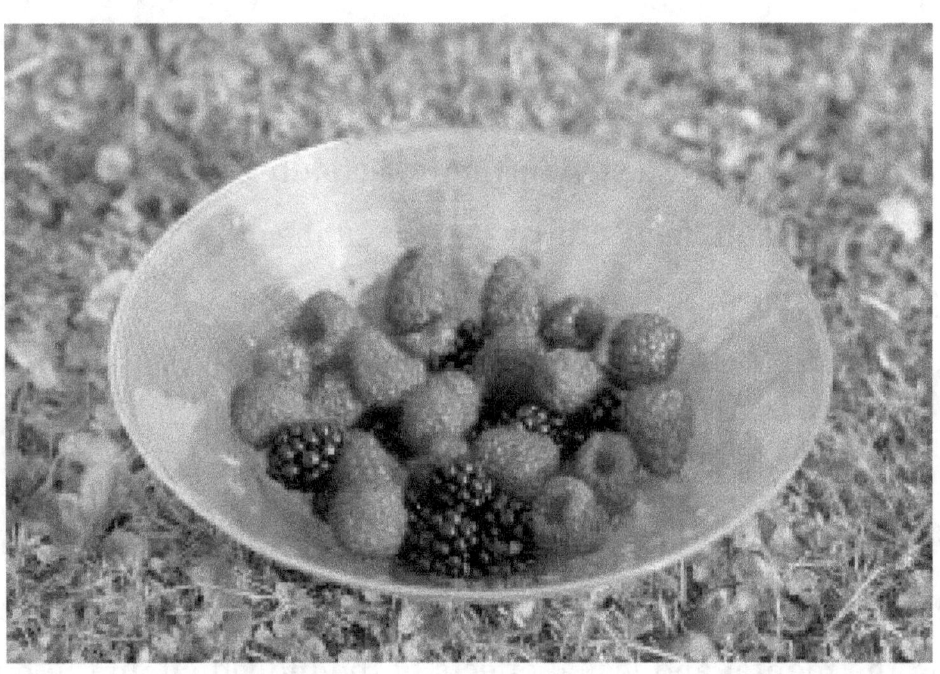

Chapter 6:

Exercise has long been advocated as an ideal way to stay healthy, next only to healthy food choices made for consumption. However for one reason or another, a lot of people do not seem to consider exercising an important part of the daily lifestyle schedule. This is an even more disastrous decision, when it is accompanied by poor diet habits.

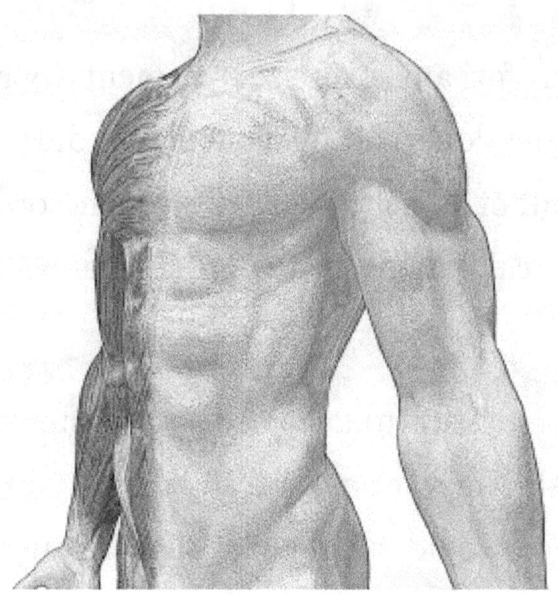

Great Info

In the quest to stay healthy through regular exercise regiments, it may be prudent to take the time to understand just how an exercise regiment can contribute positively to the overall well being of an individual. The following are just some points on how exercise can contribute to a healthier lifestyle:

Regular exercise sessions can help to keep the body weight under control thus avoiding the possibility of gaining unnecessary weight and becoming overweight.

However in order for any exercise regiment to have any positive impact, it should be done with a regular schedule in place and with the accompaniment of a healthy diet choice, and only then can it help to keep the access calories from turning into unwanted fats stored in the body.

Regular exercise also helps to keep the body systems is prime optimal working order. All the various body systems will be able to work efficiently as there would be regular dispercement of oxygen and blood flow to the various parts of the body at all times.

Mentally and physically the body will be able to functions better and be more alert.

Regular exercise has also been known to help the body produce the necessary chemical make-ups that keep a good balance within the system. This essential chemical balance can contribute positively to the avoidance of negativity in the body system, without which, symptoms such as depression and mood swings are very likely to occur.

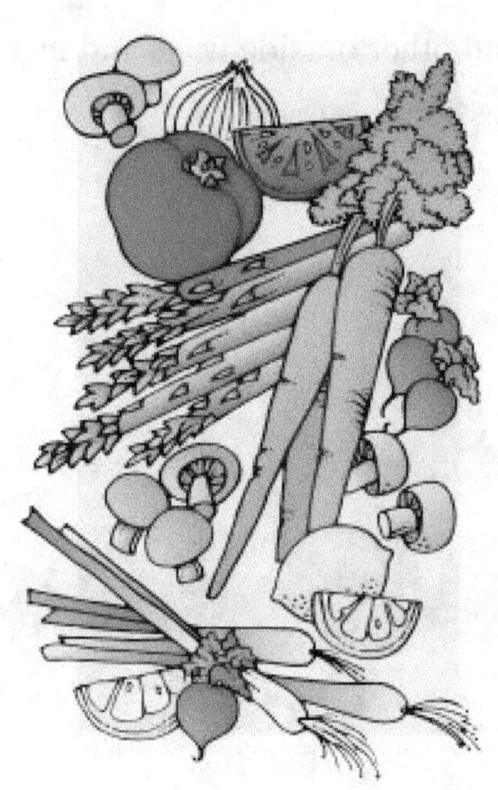

Chapter 7:
Detox Your Waste Away

The body naturally has its own detoxifying ways of getting rid of any negative residues left within the body system at regular intervals. However with the current lifestyles in place it is often difficult for the body to make such detox exercises complete and effective. Therefore there is a need to find other outside ways and means to help the body through the detox sessions.

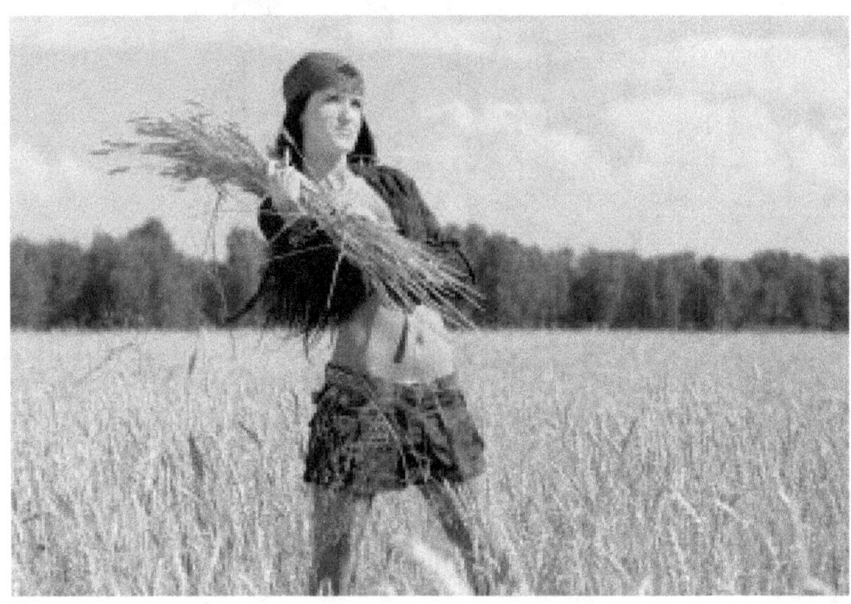

Detox

Originally meant to eradicate the body system of alcohol and drugs there are now detox programs to actually help to recreate the optimum body conditioning for compete and better health. Such programs are fast gaining popularity and if used according to instruction the resulting conditions can be very impressive indeed.

Using certain diets, herbs and other specifically designed methods these detox programs help to remove any environmental and dietary toxins from the body system. Some of the ideas behind the use of these detox programs may include minimizing the amount of chemicals ingested which can be done with the consumption of just organic foods.

Another detox exercise would be designed around choosing foods that provide optimum vitamins, nutrient and antioxidants that the body needs to launch the detoxification exercise. There is also the detox program that contains foods such as those high in fiber and water to help draw out and eliminate toxins by increasing the frequency of bowel movements and urination.

All these efforts are needed to ensure optimum health simply because most adults live a lifestyle that is not very healthy to start with, thus the need for such invasive programs to keep the healthy balance in check.

Most people who advocate the use of detox programs on a fairly regulatory schedule, attest to the overall better health conditions. These may be evident in better and clearer skin conditions, more energy, regular bowel movements, better digestion, increased levels of concentration and generally any other positive improvements felt.

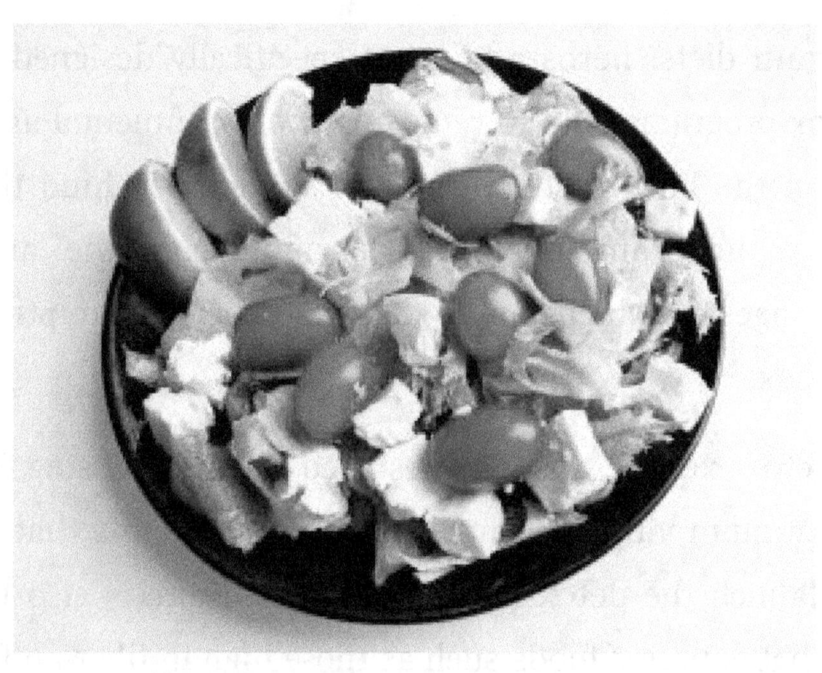

Chapter 8:
Essential Vitamins

The following is a general breakdown of the essential vitamins that would prove to be advantages to include into the diet plan for better health:

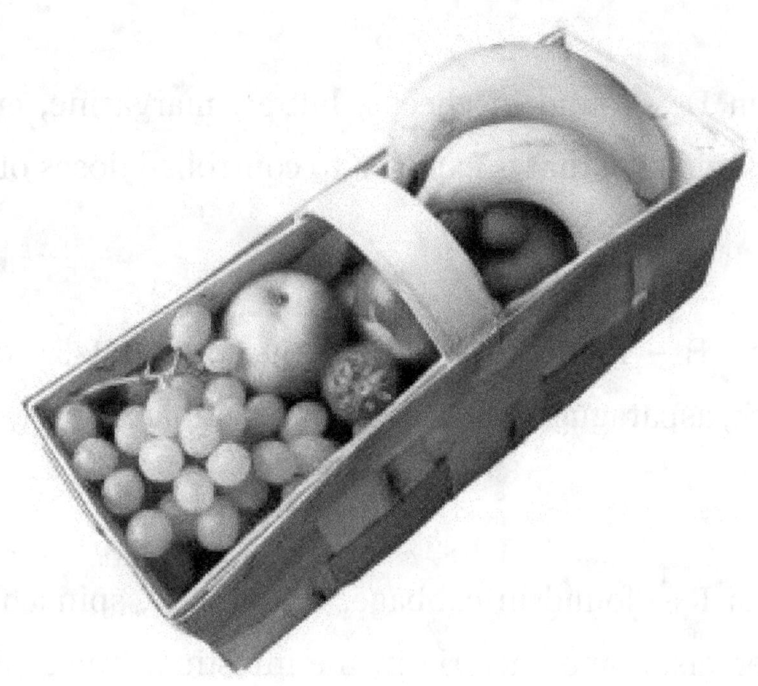

What's Needed

- Vitamin A – found in milk, cheese, cream, liver, kidney and certain types of fish oils. These have high content of saturated fats and cholesterol. Vegetable that are brighter and more vibrant in color contain higher levels of beta-carotene content.

- Vitamin D – found in cheese, butter, margarine, cream, fish, oysters and skin that is exposed to controlled doses of sunlight.

- Vitamin E – found in wheat germ, corn, nuts, seeds, olives, spinach, asparagus and other leafy vegetable and vegetable oils.

- Vitamin K – found in cabbage, cauliflower, spinach, soybeans and cereals. Some bacteria in the intestinal tracks also help to produce this vitamin.

- Thiamine also known as Vitamin B1 – found in fortifies breads, cereals, pasta, whole grains, lean meats, fish, dried beans, peas and soybeans, dairy products, certain fruits and vegetables.

- Niacin also known as Vitamin B3 – found in dairy products, poultry, fish, lean meats, nuts, legumes and enriched breads and cereals.

- Folate – found in green, leafy vegetables and many foods which are now fortified with this.

- Vitamin B12 – found in eggs, meats, poultry, shellfish and milk or milk based products.

- Pantothenic acid and biotin – found in eggs, fish, dairy products, whole grain cereals, legumes, yeast, broccoli and other vegetables in the cabbage family, white and sweet potatoes, lean beef and other similar category foods.

Wrapping Up

Optimum body functions today require any added help it can get, as most people don't take the trouble to consume foods that are healthy and beneficial to them. Therefore there is a need to make a conscious effort to source out essential vitamin types of foods and include them into the daily diet plan for hoped good health conditions.

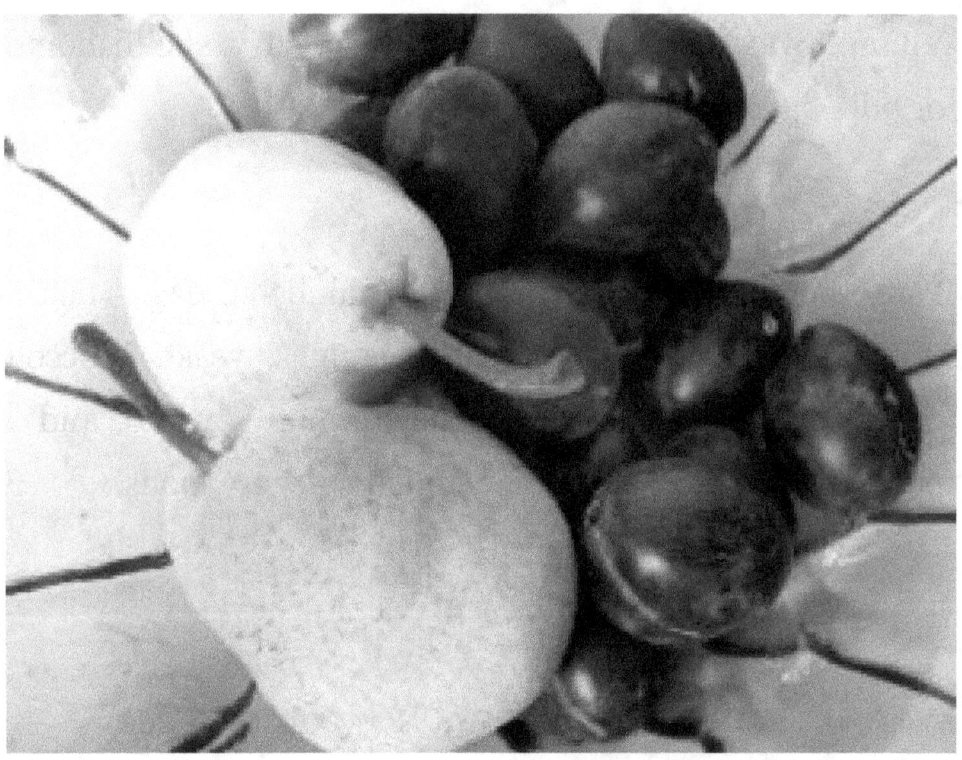

Sabat Beatto